Hormone Reset Diet
100+ Breakfast to Dessert Recipes to Boost Metabolism, Balance Hormones, and Lose Weight Fast

[Third Edition]

© **Copyright 2016 by Laura Bennett - All rights reserved.**

This document is geared towards providing exact and reliable information in regards to the topic and issue covered. The publication is sold with the idea that the publisher is not required to render accounting, officially permitted, or otherwise, qualified services. If advice is necessary, legal or professional, a practiced individual in the profession should be ordered.

- From a Declaration of Principles which was accepted and approved equally by a Committee of the American Bar Association and a Committee of Publishers and Associations.

In no way is it legal to reproduce, duplicate, or transmit any part of this document in either electronic means or in printed format. Recording of this publication is strictly prohibited and any storage of this document is not allowed unless with written permission from the publisher. All rights reserved.

The information provided herein is stated to be truthful and consistent, in that any liability, in terms of inattention or otherwise, by any usage or abuse of any policies, processes, or directions contained within is the solitary and utter responsibility of the recipient reader. Under no circumstances will any legal responsibility or blame be held against the publisher for any reparation, damages, or monetary loss due to the information herein, either directly or indirectly.

Respective authors own all copyrights not held by the publisher.

The information herein is offered for informational purposes solely, and is universal as so. The presentation of the information is without contract or any type of guarantee assurance.

The trademarks that are used are without any consent, and the publication of the trademark is without permission or backing by the trademark owner. All trademarks and brands within this book are for clarifying purposes only and are the owned by the owners themselves, not affiliated with this document.

© Copyright 2016 by   Laura Bennett   - All rights reserved.

Hormone Reset Diet

Table of Contents

Introduction	v
Chapter 1: Breakfast Recipes	1
Chapter 2: Lunch Recipes	21
Chapter 3: Dinner Recipes	44
Chapter 4: Snack and Dessert Recipes	63
Chapter 5: Smoothies Recipes	74
Conclusion	83

Introduction

Thank you for downloading the third edition of "Hormone Reset Diet: 100+ Breakfast to Dessert Recipes to Boost Metabolism, Balance Hormones, and Lose Weight Fast."

Have you ever wished that you could just turn back time? That time when you didn't had a bulging belly, most of your clothes fit, or when you had a perfect bikini body? If you had access to a magical remote that could rewind time, would you dare use it? I bet your answer would be an astounding "yes!"

Well, you can stop your wishful thinking because there is a way that you can bring back your old (ideal) body back. No, a magical remote like that from Adam Sandler's movie "Click" hasn't been invented yet. But there is a breakthrough in the health and diet world that can help individuals like you to push the reset button on their messed up hormones (Yes! Your hormones is a major factor why you're gaining weight) and return their body into a fat-burning state, instead of a fat-storing state.

If you're tired of trying all sorts of fad diets and restrictive food plans, then you've downloaded the right book. The Hormone Reset Diet is not restrictive and will not encourage you to skip meals. In fact, with this diet, you can fight weight gain with food—*the right kind of food*. The idea of this diet is to address the root cause of weight gain and that is hormonal issues. Forget about restricting calories or increasing your consumption of fat to reduce fat, weight gain and weight loss are all about hormones.

Of course, as this is a recipe book, the majority of the chapters are recipes that I'm very excited to share with you. I have expanded the previous edition of this book and added in more recipes for you. I assure you that these dishes are delicious and are very easy to follow; so you get to enjoy your weight loss journey instead of it being a drag.

I must remind you this early though, that to be able to get the results you want, it all boils down to your discipline, commitment of following the diet and embracing it as a lifestyle.

If you think you're ready to push the reset button, whip delicious dishes in your kitchen, and gain back the fantastic body you once had, jump on the next page now!

Chapter 1: Breakfast Recipes

Ah breakfast—the most important meal of the day, and yet, most of us neglect it because number one, we simply don't have time to cook and prepare and early morning meal and number two, we can just have a huge lunch since we already skipped our first meal.

Although these reasons may seem valid, but skipping breakfast might be the reason why you're lacking energy for the heavy morning grind and why you tend to overeat for the rest of the afternoon (thus the weight gain).

A study from The National Weight Loss Registry reports that individuals who eat full breakfasts for at least 5 days a week have successfully avoided gaining weight. Nutrition experts suggest that a good breakfast should contain at least 30g of protein to provide energy and fill you up througout the day. Also, when you skip breakfast, the body tends to produce more stress hormones which again, contributes to weight loss and is a risk factor for heart attacks.

If you're really serious in losing weight and being over-all healthy, then waking up early to prepare your meals for breakfast wouldn't be too much of a big deal. In this chapter, I will share with you recipes you will enjoy eating.

Oats and Chia Berry Mix

Quick, easy to make, and delicious! This recipe makes use of the superfood, chia seeds that is packed with fiber and protein. It is believed to aid in weight loss and can help you feel full much longer.

Ingredients:
¼ cup steel cut oats
1 ¼ cups water
1/8 tsp. salt
1 tsp. flax seeds, ground
2 tsp. chia seeds
1 tsp. goji berries
1/8 tsp. cinnamon powder
½ cup raspberries, frozen and then thawed
2 tbsp. raw walnuts, chopped
¼ cup plain almond milk

Steps:
1. Cook the oats with the water and salt in a sauce pan.
2. Halfway through cooking, add the flax seeds, chia seeds, goji berries, 1 tbsp. chopped walnuts and sprinkle with cinnamon power.
(Tip: If you have the spare time to prepare ahead, it is a good idea to cook large batches of oats during your free time so you can have something to re-heat and eat throughout the week)
3. Mix all the ingredients thoroughly and cook until done.
4. Before serving, pour the almond milk and then top with the remaining walnuts. Serve warm.
5. Enjoy!

Hearty Sausage and Veggie Stir-Fry

You can never go wrong with sausages for breakfast. Throw in some chopped veggies, mushrooms, and beans, *voila!* You have yourself a full and yummy meal to start the day ahead.

Ingredients:
1 lb. turkey sausage (organic is recommended)
¼ cup white kidney beans
½ cup mushrooms, chopped
½ cup yellow onion, chopped
5 cloves of garlic, chopped
2 cups chopped kale leaves
1 cup red bell pepper, chopped
½ cup zucchini, chopped
1 tbsp. Italian seasoning
Salt and pepper to taste
1 tbsp. ghee or olive oil

Steps:
1. Drizzle ghee or olive oil in skillet and heat over medium fire. Place the sausage in the heated oil and cook thoroughly.
2. Throw in the chopped onions, garlic, red bell pepper and zucchini. Cook and stir for a few minutes or until the vegetables are tender.
3. Throw in the mushrooms and then the chopped kale. Stir again for another few minutes until the kale leaves has wilted.
4. Sprinkle with salt, pepper, and Italian seasoning.
5. Serve the sausage and veggie stir-fry on top of cooked white kidney beans.
6. Enjoy!

Loaded Egg Scramble

Scrambled eggs are breakfast comfort food, but what if we level them up and load it with sautéed vegetables. Wouldn't that be amazing? Here's a delicious egg recipe you can cook and prepare in under 15 minutes.

Ingredients:
2 pcs. free-range egg
¼ cup yellow bell pepper, chopped
¼ cup green bell pepper, chopped
½ cup yellow onion, chopped
1 cup Swiss chards or kale, thinly sliced
1 tbsp. ghee or virgin coconut oil
Salt and pepper to taste
Dash of Sriracha sauce (optional)

Steps:
1. Heat the oil in a large skillet over medium fire.
2. Throw in the onion and chopped bell peppers and saute for a good 2-3 minutes.
3. Add the chopped greens and stir. Continue to cook until the leaves has just about wilted.
4. Move the cooked vegetables on one side of the pan.
5. Scramble the eggs in a bowl and pour over the other side of the pan and allow to set.
6. Once the eggs are cooked, mix it together with the sauteed vegetables.
7. Season with salt and pepper and a dash of Sriracha or any hot sauce you prefer.

Breakfast Pudding

Pudding for breakfast? Why not! This is a make-ahead recipe if you're in a rush the next day. It's heaping with nutritious super foods such as goji berries, flaxseeds, and chia seeds, and is a great fixer-upper in for an early morning grind.

Ingredients:
½ cup chia seeds
2 cups (divided) almond milk, unsweetened
1 pc. banana, chopped
¼ cup goji berries
½ tbsp. almonds, chopped
½ tbsp. flax seeds
1/8 tsp. cinnamon powder
½ tsp. vanilla extract
1/8 tsp. kosher salt

Steps:
1. In a serving bowl, combine the chia seeds, vanilla syrup, and kosher salt.
2. Pour a cup of the almond milk and stir until all the ingredients are mixed well.
3. Place in the fridge and leave it there to soak overnight.
4. For breakfast, add the remaining almond milk into the pudding. Then mix in the chopped bananas, goji berries, almonds, flax seeds, and a dash of cinnamon.
5. Stir and enjoy. (If you want your pudding warm, you can heat it up in a saucepan over low fire

Coco-Berry Pancakes

Don't you just love it when you start your day with pancakes? There's no need to worry! This recipe won't ruin your diet—it can even help curve your midday hunger and boost your energy.

The best thing that I love about this recipe besides the taste? You can cook it in just 15 minutes!

Ingredients:
1/3 cup coconut flour
½ cup blueberries
2 pcs. bananas, ripe
4 free-range eggs
1 tbsp. almond milk
1 tsp. vanilla extract
coconut oil or ghee for frying

Steps:
1. Cut the bananas in half and put it in a food processor or a blender. Add the eggs, almond milk, vanilla extract, and the coconut flour. Pulse until you achieve a smooth consistency and you are able to pour the batter.
2. Place the batter in a mixing bowl and fold in the blueberries.
3. Heat the oil in nonstick skillet over medium fire.
4. Scoop 2 to 3 spoonfuls of the batter into the hot pan and cook for 2 minutes.
5. Flip the pancakes and then cook the other side for another 2 minutes or until golden brown.
6. Repeat the process until you've finished all the batter.
7. Serve and enjoy.

Warm Garbanzo Beans Soup

From its name, you get the idea that this dish is perfect for a cold winter morning. If you love filling up your belly with something warm and hearty, you will surely love this recipe!

Ingredients:
1 cup garbanzo beans (also called as chickpeas), cooked
1 cup broccoli florets, chopped
2 pcs. celery, diced
2 cups carrots, peel removed and diced
2 cloves of garlic, chopped
½ cup onion, chopped
4 cups water
2 tbsp. coconut oil or olive oil
Kosher salt to taste

Steps:
1. Place a pot over medium heat. Drizzle the oil and then toss in the garlic and onions. Sauté for a minute and then throw in the diced celery and diced carrots.
2. Cook the veggies for about 8 minutes or until tender.
3. Add the broccoli into the pot along with the pre-cooked garbanzo beans and stir for another 2-3 minutes.
4. Pour the water, cover and bring into a boil.
5. Once boiling, reduce the heat and allow to simmer for 10 minutes or until all the veggies are tender.
6. Season with salt and transfer into 4 serving bowls.
7. Serve hot.

Guiltless Hash

Didn't I tell you earlier? You are going to love this diet (instead of dreading it) because you still get to eat yummy dishes even if you're trying to lose weight! Here's a special favorite of mine.

Just a friendly warning though, this recipe takes time to prepare and cook—but hey, it's really worth the wait!

Ingredients:
3 large sweet potatoes (organic is recommended)
2 large onions
6 cloves of garlic, minced
1 lb. Italian sausage (watch out for the sodium content!)
¼ cup rosemary (stalks removed)
1 tbsp. coconut oil or olive oil
Another 3 tbsp. of oil
A pinch of kosher salt
More salt, plus pepper to taste
Spring onion for garnish, chopped

Steps:
1. Set your oven at 450F.
2. Remove the peel from the onions and cut them in half, lengthwise. And then cut them thinly. Set aside.
3. Drizzle the 1 tbsp. oil in a pan heated over medium-high fire.
4. When the oil is hot, throw in the sliced onions and season with a pinch of salt.
5. Stir and set the fire to low. Allow the onions to sweat and caramelize for 30 minutes. Remember to stir occasionally to avoid burning.
6. Continue cooking until the onion turns dark brown.
7. While waiting for the onions to cook, place the sausages in another skillet heated over medium-high fire. Divide the sausage into smaller crumbles

and then allow to cook for 10 minutes or until it is brown and almost crisp.
8. Scoop the excess oil from the sausage.
9. While waiting for both the onions to caramelize and the sausages to brown, prepare the sweet potatoes by cutting it into cubes (about half an inch).
10. Mince the garlic and the rosemary leaves.
11. Place the sweet potato cubes in a large mixing bowl and then add the garlic and rosemary. Season with salt and pepper, and then drizzle with 3 tbsp. of oil. Toss the ingredients togethe,r making sure they are well incorporated.
12. When the oinons are caramelized and the sausages are ready, add them to the mixing bowl and stir.
13. Prepare a baking sheet by lining it with parchment paper.
14. Dump all the sweet potato and sausage mixture into the baking sheet, making sure that it is evenly distributed.
15. Place in the oven to roast for 30 to 40 minutes or until the sweet potatoes are soft and tender.
16. Remove from the oven when cooked and garnish with chopped spring onions on top.
17. Serve warm and enjoy with the whole gang.

Gingersnap Cookie Oatmeal

Are you craving for cookies yet worried about getting your diet ruined? Worry not, here is a little treat for a good one like you.

Ingredients:
1/4 cup of rolled oats (quick-cook)
1 gingersnap cookie (crushed coarsely)
1/2 cup of milk (optional)

Steps:
1. Check oats package for cooking directions and cook accordingly.
2. Sprinkle the oatmeal with crushed cookie and serve.
3. If you want to use recipe for evening snack, simply add 1/2 cup of milk.

The Omelette

We all know that eggs are healthy, but this recipe is even healthier. If you want to push it a notch higher, here is the perfect recipe for you. Both healthy and good for your hormones!

Ingredients:
1/2 cup mushrooms (sliced)
1/4 cup green bell pepper (diced)
1/4 cup red bell pepper (diced)
1/4 red onion (chopped)
1 tbsp. Olive oil (extra virgin)
1 omega-3 egg (large)
1 slice of rye toast
2 tsp. Goat cheese (crumbled)
3 egg whites (medium or large)

Steps:
1. Heat olive oil in your pan and make sure the heat is set to medium.
2. Add and saute the mushroom, onion, and peppers until soft.
3. In a small bowl, beat the egg whites and eggs until blended.
4. By this time, the vegetables are most likely soft. Transfer to a small bowl and set them aside.
5. Carefully transfer the beaten eggs into the pan.
6. Cook the beaten eggs over medium heat until set.
7. On top of the cooked egg, evenly spread the vegetables and top it with goat cheese.
8. Fold the omelette and serve with rye toast. Enjoy!

Cheese Oatmeal Pancakes

Oatmeal is healthy and it is full of fibers. Pancake is good on its own little way too. While the pancakes are usually okay, there is something that we can probably all agree to about the oatmeal. The taste is quite bland and plainly adding fruits on it sometimes do not do their magic. Now, here is a little recipe that can help spice up your morning oatmeal and give your pancakes a new kick!

Ingredients:
1/2 tsp. Vanilla extract (pure)
1/2 Ricotta or cottage cheese (low-fat)
1/4 cup of blueberries (fresh)
1 cup oats (old-fashioned, slow-cook)
1 tbsp. Flaxseed or Chia (ground)
2 tsp. Canola oil
6 egg whites

Steps:
1. In a large bowl, mix the ground seeds and oats.
2. Add the cheese, blueberries, egg whites, and vanilla extract and stir.
3. Heat the oil (canola) in a medium-sized pan over medium heat.
4. Pour the batter on the pan and wait until cooked. You will know this by seeing bubbles on the batter and the edges are hard enough to lift.
5. Flip the pancake so you can cook the other side.
6. Repeat the first five steps for the rest of the mixture.
7. Add the fresh blueberries before serving.

Skinny Waffles

Oh these lovely waffles! They would have been wonderful if only this lovely food do not make us fat. But guess what, I found a way that can help you enjoy waffles without gaining so much weight.

Ingredients:
1/4 tsp. of baking powder
1/4 cup of coconut flour
1/4 tsp. of sea salt
1 tbsp. of coconut oil
1 tbsp. of Truvia baking blend
1 tbsp. of almond milk (unsweetened)
2 tsp. of cinnamon
4 eggs (medium)
Nonstick cooking spray

Steps:
1. Prepare your waffle iron by preheating.
2. Add all the ingredients to a bowl, leaving the cooking spray.
3. Use the cooking spray on the waffle iron to glaze it.
4. Pour just half of the batter into the iron.
5. Let it cook until the batter turns golden brown.
6. Remove from the cooked waffle from the iron and repeat the previous steps for the rest of the batter.
7. Top with berries or cinnamon before serving.

Avocado Bake

Avocados are nice with sugar, but we know that as much as we can avoid drowning ourselves in sweetness, we have to. A little dash of sugar is good, but so much of it can cause you hard. So now that you are trying to avoid sugar, how can you add a little kick to your avocado now? Luckily, I stumbled upon this recipe and I'd very much like to share it with you.

Ingredients:
2 pcs. Avocados
4 eggs (large)
Feta Cheese
Green Onions
Pepper
Salt

Steps:
1. Prepare the oven and preheat to 350 degrees.
2. While waiting for the oven, vertically cut the avocados in two and remove the pit.
3. On a baking dish, place the avocado with its sliced side up.
4. Crack one egg for each avocado half and add a touch of salt and pepper.
5. Put the baking dish with avocado in the oven and let the egg bake as desired.
6. Add the feta cheese and green onions for toppings. Serve and enjoy.

Homemade Almond Milk

Want something different to start your day with, other than a glass of your traditional milk? Here is a little work around, that I lately found, for that.

Ingredients:

1 cup almonds (raw)
3 cups of cold water

Steps:
1. Prepare your blender by filling it with water.
2. Add the raw almonds and place the blender's lid.
3. Pulverize the almonds by setting it on high puree for 2 minutes.
4. Make sure that there are no chunks left in the mixture.
5. Place a straining cloth or towel on a bowl.
6. Pour the almond milk on the bowl cloth.
7. Twist the cloth and squeeze the remaining milk in the cloth or towel until all that is left on the towel are the almond pulps.
8. Store in the fridge and enjoy your almond milk!

Vanilla Raspberry Oatmeal

Being an excellent choice for breakfast, the dish provides lots of energy in the morning when you require it most.

Ingredients:
Uncooked oats: 3/4 cup
Vanilla extract: 1/2 teaspoon
Date paste: 1 tablespoon
Almond milk: 1/2 cup of
Protein powder: 1/2 scoop
Salt: A pinch
Water

Steps:
1. Mix all 7 ingredients in a bowl
2. Keep in refrigerator overnight
3. Serve cold

Tips: Serve the dish with fresh raspberries and sliced almonds (optional)

Easy Almond Milk

Why buy almond milk in the store when you can make your own healthier version at home?

Ingredients:
Raw almonds: 1/2 cup
Medjool dates: 3/4, pitted
Cinnamon: 1/2 teaspoon (optional)
Purified water: 5 cups
Pink Himalayan salt: a pinch (optional)

Steps:
1. Place water and almonds into a blender; blend on high.
2. Remove the mixture from blender when thoroughly blended; transfer into a nut milk bag.
3. Hold the bag over a bowl; squeeze the liquid mixture into the bowl from the bag.
4. Stop squeezing when until there's only pulp left in the nut milk bag; discard the pulp and transfer the strained liquid back into the blender.
5. Add cinnamon, salt and dates in the blender and blend until smooth.

Rosemary Eggs

Eggs on toasted bread are go-to comfort food, a meal to be eaten alone on a spring morning, sitting on the couch with a book, or standing up in the kitchen.

Ingredients:
Eggs: 2
Manna from heaven bread (toasted): 2 slices
Ripe avocado: 1, peel on, chopped & seeds removed
Avocado oil: 1 teaspoon

Cream cheese (low-fat): 3 tablespoons
Fresh rosemary: 1/2 teaspoon, chopped
Fresh lemon juice: 1 tablespoon
Flax oil: 1 teaspoon
Cayenne: A pinch
Salt

Steps:
1. Use a fork to mix the cheese, avocado oil, salt, fresh rosemary, lemon juice, flax oil and a pinch of cayenne on a bowl and set aside.
2. Boil two inches of water in a deep pan; then bring to simmer.
3. Place the cracked eggs in a cup one at a time and mix; pour the egg mixture very slowly into the simmering water, keeping close to the surface.
4. Simmer the eggs for 5 minutes; use a slotted spoon to remove the eggs; use excess water to drain off.
5. Spoon the chopped avocado onto toasted bread, top with the cheese mixture and poached eggs.

Orange polentina

Polentina, a creamier, porridge-like version of polenta is often served for a nutrition-rich delicious breakfast. The yogurt and tangy mascarpone cheese along with orange-infused dollop serves as a rich, delicious topping. You can save calories by doubling the yogurt and skipping the mascarpone.

Ingredients:
Orange: 1
Honey: 4 tablespoons
Mascarpone: ¼ cup
Polenta, instant: ¾ cup
Salt: ¼ teaspoon
Water: 2 cup
Milk: 1 ½ cup
Greek yogurt: ¼ cup
Chopped tarragon: 1 teaspoon

Steps:
1. Zest the orange to get around 1 ½ teaspoons. Set aside.
2. Use a sharp knife to discard the white pith and rest of the peel; separate the segments from their surrounding membranes and set aside to use as garnish.
3. Boil water along with salt and milk in a large saucepan; whisk in polenta slowly and bring it to boil again. Then maintain an even bubble by reducing the heat to medium-low; whisk for 1-5 minutes until the polentina thickens. Remove from heat; let sit, covered, for 5 minutes.
4. While the polentina is setting, combine yogurt, orange zest (½ teaspoon), honey (1 tablespoon) and mascarpone together in a small bowl.
5. When the polentina is done, whisk in the remaining zest and honey; divide among four bowls; pour a dollop of the yogurt topping.
6. Use the reserved orange segments to garnish; sprinkle with tarragon and serve right away.

Kale juice and nut

Being high in fiber and healthy protein, this dish will serve you as a wholesome breakfast.

Ingredients:
Kale juice: 1 cup
Almond, chestnut, brazil nuts: 1/2 cup
Whey protein: 1/2 cup

Steps:
Boil kale juice along with whey protein, remove from heat when it attains a thick consistency. Add almond, chestnut, and Brazil nut to it.

Breakfast soup

This soup is the solid proof that your dinner leftovers can make an excellent, high-protein breakfast!

Ingredients:
Ripe avocados: 2, peeled and pitted
Ground ginger: ½ teaspoon
Ground turmeric: ½ teaspoon
Organic chicken or vegetable broth: 1 quart
Chicken breasts: 2, cooked and diced, or
Tempeh (1 package)/ cannellini beans (1 cup) if you use vegetable broth

Steps:
1. Place broth, turmeric and avocado in a blender; blend until smooth; transfer in a 2-quart saucepan.
2. Add the ginger and chicken; heat until warm.

Apple chicken sausage

These simple, healthy sausages taste excellent, and they make an elegant breakfast or brunch dish.

Ingredients:
Diced onion: 1
Ground pepper: ¼ teaspoon
Salt: ¾ teaspoon
Chicken: 1 pounds
Apple: 1
Canola oil: 2 teaspoons
Chopped sage: 1 tablespoon
Organic honey: ½ tablespoon
Fennel seed: ½ teaspoon

Steps:
1. Heat oil in a skillet; & cook onion until begins to soften, for 2 minutes.
2. Add the apples and cook for 2 more minutes.
3. Transfer to a bowl; let sit for around 5 minutes to cool.
4. Add salt, sugar, chicken, sage, fennel and pepper into the bowl; toss gently to combine.
5. Place the mixture back into the skillet, arranging them in four flattened portions in the shape of patties.
6. Cook for 3 minutes on each side until cooked through.
7. Repeat the steps to make patties with the whole mixture.

Chapter 2: Lunch Recipes

After a filling breakfast you surely wouldn't need to eat a heavy lunch. So in this chapter, you will mostly find light and healthy midday meals which you will surely would love to devour.

Keep in mind that the goal in this diet is to get the right type of food, therefore you should expect to eat a lot of "clean" foods for your main meals.

Here are some of the recipes I gathered for lunch:

Salad Express

This recipe is plain and simple that you can prepare in a jiffy. I surely recommend this salad when you're rushing to work and have no time to cook your lunch. I promise you, even if you're a newbie in the kitchen, you will still perfect this recipe.

Ingredients:
1 pc. palm-sized cooked chicken fillet (breast part), sliced into bite-sized pieces
If you have left over chicken or fish last night, then great! You could use that to add to this salad.
2 cups of your favorite greens like kale, lettuce, or even broccoli
¼ cup cherry tomatoes, sliced in half
½ cup canned kidney beans, rinsed and drained
1 tbsp. balsamic vinegar
1 tbsp. extra virgin olive oil

Steps:
1. Whip the balsamic vinegar and olive oil in a salad bowl.

2. Throw in the chopped greens, tomatoes, and beans into the bowl and toss gently to coat with the dressing.
3. Top with the sliced chicken or fish.
4. Pack to go or enjoy the salad immediately.

Minty Chicken Skewers

BBQs are perfect for the weekend aren't they? This is a basic chicken kebob recipe with a minty dressing. Take note that this is a make-ahead dish so if you want to have this during the weekdays, it's best to prepare it the night before or the weekend before as it requires time for marinating.
Serve this dish with mixed greens or cooked quinoa on the side and you have yourself a plate rich in nutrients such as protein and B vitamins.

Ingredients:
3 pcs. chicken breasts, deboned and cut into chunks
Keep in mind that organic produce is always recommended
2 pcs. large zucchinis, cut into cubes
1 cup grape tomatoes

For the dressing:
½ cup fresh mint leaves
½ cup lemon juice
4 cloves of garlic, peel removed
1 pc. small shallot
1 tsp. kosher salt
1 tsp. crushed pepper
¾ cup extra virgin olive oil

Steps:
1. Prepare the dressing first by placing all the ingredients (except the oil) in a food processor or a blender. Pulse for 2 minutes or until you achieve a smooth consistency.
2. Continue to blend the ingredients and then slowly pour the olive oil in the mixture. Make sure to incorporate everything before turning off the food processor. Set aside.
3. Prepare the kebobs by alternately skewing the chicken and vegetables on bamboo sticks.

4. Place the kebobs in a baking dish and then poor over the mint dressing.
5. Turn the skewers to make sure it is coated with the dressing. Cover and then place in the fridge to marinate for at least 30 minutes.
6. When you're ready to cook, set the grill into medium-high and then cook the kebobs for 12-15 minutes, turning it 2 to 3 times when grilling.
7. Enjoy!

Cauli and Broccoli Salad

Here's another salad recipe I'd love to share with you. This dish contains cauliflower and broccoli which, makes it a super nutritious lunch.

Other than making you feel full after eating this meal, did you know that these cruciferous vegetables are great sources of Vitamin C and K? Plus, they also contain a compound called *glucosinolates* that is seen to reduce the risk of developing cancer.

Ingredients:
1 head cauliflower, stems removed
2 cups broccoli florets
1 large carrot, roughly chopped
½ cup parsley, chopped fine
½ cup red grapes, sliced in half
½ cup sunflower seeds
4 tbsp. freshly squeezed lemon juice
Salt and pepper to taste

Steps:
1. Thoroughly clean the broccoli and cauliflower florets.
2. Place them in a food processor and pulse until they are finely chopped. You can also do this by hand if you think you're good with your knife skills.
3. Transfer the chopped vegetables in a large bowl.
4. Add the carrots in the food processor and then pulse until it is also finely chopped. And then transfer it into the bowl with the two other veggies.
5. Throw in the sunflower seeds, parsley, and grapes in to the bowl and drizzle with the lemon juice.
6. Season with salt and pepper and then toss to mix all the ingredients together.
7. Serve and consume immediately.

Zucchini in Pesto Sauce

This is a full-vegan, pasta-like recipe as it makes use of zucchini instead of the carb-rich spaghetti. If you're trying to lose weight and wanting to heal your hormones, this is a nutritious go-to lunch for you.

Ingredients:
5 pcs. medium-sized zucchini
1 pc. ripe avocado
2 cups fresh basil leaves
1 cup arugula leaves
4 pcs. sage
1 clove of garlic
¼ cup pine nuts
2 tbsp. freshly squeezed lemon juice

Steps:
1. Wash the zucchinis thoroughly and then cut the ends.
2. Process the zucchini in a spiralizer to turn it into a pasta-like shape and set aside.
3. Prepare the pesto sauce by adding the avocado, basil leaves, arugula, sage, garlic, and pine nuts in a food processor or blender.
4. Drizzle the lemon juice and then process until you achieve a smooth consistency.
5. Pour the sauce on the prepared zucchini "pasta" and toss, making sure it is well coated with the pesto.
6. Serve and enjoy.

Sprouts and Greens Salad

Want an easy-to-make salad? If you're not intimidated by eating too many greens, then this recipe is for you. It's dressing tangy and making it is no sweat. Here's how you prepare it...

Ingredients:
2 cups baby spinach
1 cup mustard greens
1 cup kale
½ cup cilantro
½ cup alfalfa sprouts
(you can also add edible flowers like marigolds, if you like)
1 small cucumber, chopped
1 pc. carrot, grated
½ ripe avocado, cut into chunks.
¼ tsp. toasted sesame seeds and cumin, ground

For the dressing:
2 tbsp. macadamia oil
1 tsp. tahini
2 tbsp. freshly squeezed lemon juice
Pinch of kosher salt to taste

Steps:
1. Thoroughly clean your greens and sprouts and then dry them.
2. Snip the greens using a clean kitchen knife to cut them into bite-sized pieces.
3. Throw the greens and sprouts into a salad bowl and then add on top the chopped cucumber, grated carrot, and avocado chunks. Sprinkle with the sesame seeds and ground cumin mixture.
4. Whisk the ingredients for the dressing, making sure they are well mixed, and then pour over the salad.
5. For added protein, you can serve this salad with sliced hard boiled eggs on top.

Chicken and Squash Toss

The sweetness of the squash plus the tasty chicken—what else could you ask for?
Did you know that eating squash, such as butternut squash is found to help you lose weight? That's because it is low in calories and is a good source of dietary fiber so it cuts off the extra calories you usually consume for your meals.

Ingredients:
1 ½ lb. butternut squash, peel and seeds removed and then diced
1 pc. chicken breast fillet, cooked and then cut into cubes
3 cups baby spinach or any green leafy veggies of your choice
½ cup garbanzo beans (also known as chickpeas)
½ cup unsalted pistachios, chopped
2 tbsp. olive oil
Kosher salt and pepper to taste

For the dressing:
3 tbsp. extra virgin olive oil
1 tsp. Dijon mustard
2 tbsp. red wine vinegar
½ shallot, minced
Kosher salt and pepper to taste

Steps:
1. Set the oven at 400F.
2. Place the diced squash on a baking sheet and then drizzle with the 2 tbsp. olive oil.
3. Season the squash with salt and pepper and toss making sure it is well coated with the oil.
4. Place in the oven to roast for 30 minutes. Remember to give it a toss halfway through roasting so that it cooks evenly.
5. When done roasting, take out of the oven and allow to cool to room temperature.

6. While waiting for the squash to cool, whip up the dressing by whisking all the ingredients together. It is a good idea to pour the salad dressing in a resalable container such as a mason jar so you can keep the leftover in the fridge for future use.
7. When the squash is ready, transfer it in a large salad bowl and then add the baby spinach, garbanzo, pistachio, and cooked chicken cubes.
8. Drizzle with the prepared dressing and toss to coat the veggies evenly.
9. Enjoy!

Salmon Flakes Salad

As we all know, salmon is a great ingredient for your meals. It is an ideal source of protein and is also rich in omega-3 fatty acids, which helps promote our body's overall health. Take note that if you're buying salmon, it's better to choose wild caught than farm-raised as the former provides significantly more omega-3 than the latter.

Ingredients:
1 pc. large salmon fillet (wild-caught is recommended)
1 cup fresh arugula
2 pcs. artichoke hearts, chopped
10 pcs. grape tomatoes, cut in half
4 sprigs of fresh thyme
2 cloves of garlic, minced
2 tbsp. coconut oil or olive oil
Kosher salt and pepper to taste

For the dressing:
4 tbsp. extra virgin olive oil
2 tbsp. lemon juice
1 tbsp. Dijon mustard
Kosher salt and pepper to taste

Steps:
1. Pre-heat the grill on medium-low temperature.
2. Generously season the fish fillet with salt and pepper and then place on top of an aluminum foil.
3. Drizzle the fillet with the 2 tbsp. coconut oil and then season with the minced garlic and the fresh thyme on top.
4. Completely cover the salmon with the foil and grill for at least 15 minutes or until the salmon turns into a light pink and is flaky.
5. While waiting for the fish to cook, prepare the salad by tossing the arugula, chopped artichoke hearts and tomatoes in a large bowl.
6. Whisk the ingredients of the dressing together and pour over the salad. Toss well to coat the veggies with the vinaigrette. Set aside.
7. When the salmon is cooked, allow it to cool for a few minutes before pulling the fish apart into flakes using a fork.
8. Place the grilled salmon flakes on top of the salad and serve.
9. Enjoy.

Shrimp Ceviche

This dish is a healthy and light appetizer or lunch.

Ingredients:
Extra virgin olive oil: 4 tablespoons
Chopped fresh cilantro: 1/2 Cup
Garlic: 1 clove, minced
Green onions: 1 Bunch, chopped
Fresh lime juice: 3/4 Cup
Uncooked medium shrimp (peeled): 1 ½ pounds
Grated lime peel: 1 tablespoon
Serrano chili: 1, finely chopped with seeds

Diced tomatoes: 1 -2 Cups
Diced Jicama: 3/4 Cup
Avocado: 1, diced
Lime
Lemon wedges

Steps:
1. Heat the olive oil (2 tablespoons) over medium heat in large skillet; add the shrimp with pepper and salt; sauté shrimp for about 3 minutes 'till just opaque in center; transfer to large bowl, scraping up any browned bits with a wooden spoon.
2. Add lime peel and lime juice to skillet; pour over shrimp in bowl; add the remaining olive oil, chili, onion and garlic; stir to blend. Allow the mixture to stand for 30 minutes.
3. Once the shrimp is marinated, add cilantro and tomatoes. Cover and keep in fridge for 1-2 hours.
4. Add jicama, avocado and a wedge of lemon and lime.

Tomato Borscht

In this dish, you'll find almost everything you require during the middle of the day.

Ingredients:
Olive Oil: 2 Tablespoons
Vegetable Stock: 1 Pint
Tomato Juice: 8 fluid Ounces
Chopped sun-Dried Tomatoes: 1 tablespoon
Cinnamon: 1/4 teaspoon, ground
Raw Beetroot: 8 ounces, peeled & grated
Onion: 1 Small Sized, chopped
Garlic: 1 Clove, chopped
Toasted Cumin Seeds (ground): 1 teaspoon
Ripe Fresh Tomatoes: 8 ounces, chopped
Ground Black Pepper
Salt

Light Soy Sauce: 1 tablespoon
Soured Cream
Toasted Cumin Seeds

Steps:
5. Cook the olive oil, garlic and onions in a heavy pan.
6. After 5 minutes, add the beetroot.
7. When browned, add everything else except for the last 3 ingredients from list; cook for around 15 minutes.
8. Finally, add the soy sauce, soured cream and cumin seeds; serve chilled or warm.

Chicken Kabobs

Marinated in a mixture of lime and tamari sauce, these loaded skewers make for a tasty diet lunch. You can have this dish with steamed veggies or fresh salad on the side.

Ingredients:
Organic chicken breast halves (skinless, boneless): 4, cut into large chunks
Lime: 1, juiced
Tamari: 3 tablespoons
Extra virgin olive oil: 1-tablespoon
Minced garlic: 1 teaspoon
Cilantro, chopped

Steps:
9. Combine the oil, cilantro, Tamari sauce, lime juice and garlic in a small bowl.
10. Soak bamboo sticks in water for 5 minutes; skewer the chicken chunks onto the soaked bamboo sticks; marinate for at least 30 minutes.
11. Grill for 6-8 minutes on each side on medium high heat.
12. Remove from heat when the juices run clear.

Potato Pancakes

These pancakes can be eaten as a side dish to a meaty main dish, or as a meal all by themselves.

Ingredients:
Egg whites: 4
Parsley flakes: 1 tablespoon
Onion: ¼ cup, grated
Potatoes: 2 medium, cooked, peeled & grated
Plain yogurt (low-fat): ½ cup
Whole wheat flour: 1 tablespoon
Pepper
Extra virgin coconut oil (optional)

Steps:
1. Place eggs whites and potatoes into medium bowl.
2. Add the rest ingredients; mix well.
3. Heat skillet; pan fry potato cakes, flipping over. Make sure to brown them evenly on both sides.

Quick Quiche

These tempting pies prove that there are countless variations to dish up. Served on a elegant pie plate, these dishes are springtime showstoppers.

Ingredients:
Eggs: 10, beaten well
Diced ham: 4 ounces
Swiss cheese: 8oz
Diced onion: ½ cup
Water: 2tablespoons
Salt
Pepper

Steps:
1. Mix ingredients; pour into greased dish.
2. Bake for around 35-45 minutes at 375°F; remove from oven when knife comes out of center clean.

Green Salad

This dish is incredibly simple to prepare, you must give it a go. If nothing else, it can provide you some chopping skill, so why not prepare something tasty while you are practicing your knife skills?

Ingredients:
Avocado: ½, peeled & pitted
Nonfat buttermilk: ¾ cup
Fresh herbs: 2 tablespoons (e.g. Sorrel, tarragon and/or chives), chopped
Canned artichoke hearts: 1 cup, rinsed & chopped
Celery: 1/2 cup, chopped
Green leaf lettuce (bite-size pieces): 8 cups
Cucumber: ½, sliced
White-wine vinegar: 2 teaspoons
Anchovy paste: 1-teaspoon
Cooked shrimp: 12 ounces, peeled & deveined
Cherry or grape tomatoes: 1 cup
Canned chickpeas: 1 cup, rinsed

Steps:
1. Blend buttermilk, anchovy, avocado vinegar and herbs in a blender until smooth.
2. Divide lettuce among 4 plates; place cucumber, chickpeas, celery, shrimp, tomatoes and artichoke hearts on top. Pour the dressing over the salads.

Zucchini Pasta & Chicken Meatballs

Are you thinking of what else you can do with zucchini? Here is a little recipe where you can practice your pasta making skills, without actually having to eat pasta.

Ingredients:
1/2 tsp. basil (dried)
1/2 onion (medium, finely chopped)
1/4 cup of almond meal
1/4 cup of cheese
1/4 cup parsley (fresh)
1/4 tsp. of Worcestershire sauce (gluten-free)
3/4 sea salt (Celtic)
2 tbsp. of olive oil
2 lbs. Organic chicken (ground)
3 minced garlic cloves
3 zucchini (made into strips)
Tomato sauce

Steps:
1. Mix all nine ingredients in a bowl, leaving olive oil, tomato sauce and zucchini behind.
2. Make 1 1/2 inch size meatballs out of the chicken mixture by rolling them.
3. Heat the olive oil in a pan.
4. Once the pan is ready, add the meatballs. Let them brown on all sides and caramelize.
5. Add tomato sauce into the pan.
6. Carefully add the meatballs into a baking dish and cover the zucchini pasta with sauce.
7. Bake on 325 degrees.
8. Boil Zucchini strips (pasta) for 2-4 minutes, then drain.
9. Pour tomato sauce and add some meatballs.
Saute until the dish is warm and serve. Enjoy!

Hormone Reset Diet

Mac and Cheese Prosciutto with Caramelized Onion

Ingredients:
1/2 cup Parmesan cheese (grated)
1/4 tsp. of black pepper
1/4 cup of goat cheese
1 clean and trimmed head of cauliflower head
1 cup of heavy cream
1 medium diced onion
1 cup of sharp shredded cheddar cheese
2 tbsp. of olive oil
3 cloves of garlic (large, minced)
4 tbsp. of butter
6 oz. of diced Prosciutto (cooked until crisp)

Steps:
1. Preheat the oven to 350 degrees.
2. Add water about an inch high in a big pot with cover.
3. Add the cauliflower in the pot and steam until tender.
4. Once the cauliflower is tender, remove the pot from the heat.
5. Drain the water and do not remove the cauliflower in the pot yet to release the excess water.
6. Transfer cauliflower in a dish and gently break the cauliflower apart, using a fork.
7. Place a pan over medium heat.
8. Heat the olive oil and half of the butter in the pan.
9. Add the onions.
10. Saute until the mixture takes the color of caramel.
11. Remove the onions from the and set aside.
12. Add the garlic and the remaining half of butter in the pan that you used for the onions.
13. Saute until you can smell the garlic and the butter melts.
14. Add the parmesan cheese and heavy cream.
15. Stir until the parmesan melts and let the sauce boil.
16. Add the black pepper, cheddar cheese, and goat cheese.

17. Mix until the cheese melts and blends in the sauce nicely.
18. Lower the heat. Simmer for 5 minutes and let the sauce thicken.
19. Pour the cheese and let it evenly cover the cauliflower.
20. Add the caramelized onions on top of the cheese sauce.
21. Add the prosciutto on top of the onions.
22. Sprinkle the rest of the cheese that you did not melt.
23. Place in the oven and let it bake for 15 minutes.
24. Serve and enjoy!

Cordon Bleu Casserole

The love of chicken, cheese and ham. Are you craving for it yet worried on how to replace it with healthier options and still get that sumptuous flavor? Worry not anymore! Here is a recipe that can give you your cordon bleu craving!

Ingredients:
1/2 cup of broth (chicken)
1/2 cup of sour cream
1 lb. Cubed chicken breast (trimmed of fat)
1 head of cauliflower (large, cleaned and trimmed)
1 cup of grated parmesan cheese (divided)
1 tsp. of tarragon
1 1/4 cup of heavy cream
3 tbsp. of salted butter
3 oz. of chopped mushrooms
3.5 oz. swiss cheese (must be divided)
4 oz. of chopped onion
12 oz. diced ham
Pepper
Salt

Steps:
Start with having the oven preheated to 350 degrees.

25. Place a large pan over medium heat and let the chicken and butter cook in it.
26. Let the chicken turn brown on both sides.
27. Once done, add the onion, mushrooms, and ham. Reduce the heat.
28. Let the onion turn translucent.
29. In another pot with cover, place the cauliflower head in chicken broth.
30. Steam until tender and drain the broth, leaving the cauliflower to let the excess water out.
31. Once excess water is out, mash the cauliflower with fork.
32. Combine the parmesan cheese, heavy cream, swiss cheese, salt, tarragon, and pepper in a bowl over medium to high heat.
33. Let it boil and once done, reduce the heat to low.
34. Simmer for 10 minutes and do not forget to frequently stir.
35. Once done, combine the cauliflower, sauce, and meat.
36. Cover the top of the mixture with parmessan and swiss cheese.
37. Put in the oven and bake it for 25 minutes.

Spinach and Kale Pie

Spinach and kale, with some cheese isn't a bad idea at all, isn't it? Do you want to have it for lunch? That's one good pie to turn your cravings too, instead of eating pizza which is packed with tons of oil, carbohydrates and sky-rocketing calorie amount. Here's a recipe to save your lunch.

NOTE: If you want to make a quiche pie, make sure to brush butter into the crust before putting in the egg mix.

Ingredients:
1 chopped fresh spinach
1 cup of chopped kale
1 1/2 cups cream
3/4 gruyere cheese
3/4 cheddar cheese
2 diced shallots, preferable sauted either using bacon or butter
10 pcs. Cooked to crisp bacon (sliced)
Sea salt
Ground pepper

Steps:
Get the thawed pie crust and heat it to 375 in the oven.

38. Start frying the bacon, and while waiting for it to go crispy.
39. Mix both eggs and cream and beat it till thoroughly mixed.
40. Add in a pinch of salt and small amount of fresh ground pepper into the bowl.
41. Begin chopping all the vegetables. Grate the two cheese and check the bacon if it is already cooked.
42. Add the shallots on the pan.
43. Sautee it together for an additional 5 minutes.
44. Lifting the bacon off the pan before it gets burned.
45. Place both the shallots and bacon on kitchen towel to soak on excess oil and fat.
46. Place the sliced bacon, vegetable and cheese into the mixed egg and cream.
47. Once thoroughly mixed, pour it carefully onto the crust from the oven.
48. Bake in the oven again for 40-45minutes more. You can also set aside the quiche spills not to waste the excess by preparing a cookie sheet and tray for it to be placed on later
49. Let it all cool until is warm enough to serve.

Glazed Tomato and Turkey Curry Meatloaf

Who wants meatloaf and curry? What if we put them together and make a nice lunch out of them, huh? Below is a recipe for a nice, hormone resetting lunch for you!

Ingredients:
2 tbsp. Minced garlic
3/4 cup oats (rolled)
1 can roasted tomatoes (diced and strained)
1 tbsp olive oil (extra virgin)
1 lb turkey (ground, dark meat)
1/2 cup water or chicken stock
1/2 zucchini (grated)
Salt (kosher)
Ground Pepper (fresh)
1 pc. Egg, whisked lightly
3 tbsp. Maple syrup (pure)
2 tbsp. Powdered curry mix
3 tbsp. Apricots (dried and chopped)
3 tbsp. Pistachios (whole)

Steps for Sauce:

50. Make a puree out of the tomatoes, pouring it together with the chicken stock into a blender until it is consistently smooth.
51. Get a saucepan, warm in medium heat with olive oil. Sautee with garlic for at least a minute.
52. Evenly stir the maple syrup with the pureed tomato.

53. Add salt (kesher type) and twist some ground pepper. Let it sit on low heat for 5 minutes with pan uncovered. Once done, put it out of the stove and let it cool down and go onto the preparation of the turkey mix.

Steps for the Meatloaf:

1. Set oven for 375 F.
2. Lay down parchment paper with baking sheet.
3. Mix ingredients in a large bowl. Add in the previously mixed tomato sauce a while back.
4. Mix ingredients by hand, make sure it is thoroughly and evenly dispersed. Do not overknead.
5. Place it in to the baking sheet, shaping the loaf. Drizzle a bit of olive oil again then put it again in the oven for 30 minutes more.
6. Grab the remainder of the sauce made and pour it completely on top of the load, then roast for 15 more minutes.
7. Put it out of the oven, let it cool down for 10 minutes. Slice it evenly and serve it with the sauce.

Roasted Salmon with Beets

It's been suggested that we should never be afraid of stuffing ourselves with salmon for at least every two days. That means needing a couple of recipes so as not to get bored with it. Here is a salmon recipe to help you out!

Ingredients:
1 ½ pound salmon fillet (skinless)
1 tbsp fresh chives (chopped finely)
1 tbsp terragon (chopped finely)
1 tbsp fresh parsley; flat leaf (chopped finely)
4 (1 pound) beets; medium and golden (preferred); thinly lengthwise sliced
6 tbsp olive oil (extra virgin)
1 tbsp lemon zest (grated)
4 cups baby greens (mixed)
3 tbsp shallots (finely chopped)
¼ cup lemon juice (fresh)
1 pinch salt (kosher)
1 pinch black pepper (ground; fresh)

Steps:
1. Prepare the oven. It should be preheated to 450 degrees.
2. Grab a baking sheet.
3. Coat the beets onto 1 ½ tablespoons of olive oil. Add some salt and pepper for seasoning. P
4. lace the beets onto the center of the baking sheet, making way for the salmon as the top part while beets as the bed.
5. Cook the beets for 20 minutes until it roasted to tender crisp.
6. Put the salmon above the beets. Again, brush ½ tablespoon of oil to the salmon and season with salt and pepper.
7. Mix the parsley chives and tarragon in a large bowl. Place a tablespoon of the mixture on top of the salmon.

8. Place it in the oven for another 15 minutes. Check to see that it should be cooked by medium rare doneness to have a slightly rosy center. Remove it out of the oven.
9. Spread the remaining 4 tablesppons of oil, shallots, lemon zest and lemon juice onto the herbs. Season it with salt and pepper.
10. Make a salad out of the mixed greens with 2 tablespoons of the homemade dressing. Sprinkle the dressing all throughout the salmon and beets. Serve the greens on the side.

Chapter 3: Dinner Recipes

You've worked so hard throughout the day, so you deserve a good meal before you call it a night. As I've said this type of diet isn't restrictive at all as long as your meals are made of whole and nutritious ingredients. In this chapter I will share with you recipes for main meals, like dinner.

Ground Turkey on Lettuce Cups

I enjoy making this recipe when I'm too lazy to cook. As you may have already figured out, the hormone reset diet would require you to prepare and cook your food more than buying something from a restaurant.
This is important as you want to keep watch over what you put on your plate. This recipe is a favorite of mine because it is easy to make and much easier to eat.

Ingredients:
½ lb. turkey, ground
1 can (15 oz.) black beans, rinsed and drained
½ cup fresh cilantro, chopped
½ cup onion, chopped
¼ tsp. garlic powder
A pinch of red pepper flakes
¼ tsp. chili powder
Kosher salt and pepper to taste
8-10 pcs. iceberg lettuce cups
1 medium sized tomato, chopped
Spring onion for garnish, chopped
½ lime cut into wedges
2 tbsp. olive oil or ghee

Steps:
1. Drizzle the olive oil into a skillet and heat over medium fire.

2. When the oil is hot, sauté the onions for a minute and then add the ground turkey.
3. Stir and season with salt and pepper. Also add the garlic powder, red pepper flakes, and chili powder. Stir well.
4. Continue cooking until the ground turkey is cooked through.
5. Throw in the black beans and cilantro into the pan. Stir and allow to heat for a minute or two and turn off the heat.
6. Place the lettuce cups in a serving plate and then top it with the prepared ground turkey and beans and then garnish with the chopped tomato and spring onion.
7. Serve with the lemon wedge on the side. Enjoy!

Slow-Cooked Pulled Pork

Don't have time to make a proper dinner? Here's a recipe you can place in the crock-pot and then leave it to cook for a few hours. Isn't that just perfect?

Ingredients:
1 lb. pork roast
½ onion, sliced
1 large tomato, peeled and then diced
1 can green chili
¼ tsp. chili powder
¼ tsp. garlic powder
Kosher salt and pepper to taste

Steps:
1. Place the pork roast at the bottom of the crock pot and then followed by all the ingredients.
2. Set the slow cooker on low and leave it cook for at least 7 hours.
3. When you're done cooking, remove the pork from the pot and then shred it using a fork.

4. You can serve this on top of mixed greens or a whole-wheat tortilla.
5. Enjoy!

Yummy Crab Cakes

Did you know that crabs contain what is called *chitosan* which is known to naturally block fat. What a perfect fat-busting recipes is this? Do you agree?

Ingredients:
½ lb. crab meat, cooked
2 free-range eggs
4 pcs. radishes, cut into smaller pieces
1 clove of garlic
1 pc shallot
½ tsp. garlic powder
½ tsp. smoked paprika
1 tsp. dried parsley
Kosher salt and pepper to taste
3 tbsp. olive oil

Steps:
1. Place the radish, garlic, and shallot in a food processor and pulse until they are minced.
2. In a large bowl, whisk the eggs and then add the minced ingredients in the same bowl.
3. Also add the crab meat along with the garlic powder, paprika, parsley, and season with salt and pepper. Using your hands, thoroughly mix the ingredients together and then forming them into small, flat patties.
4. Heat the olive oil in a frying pan and then place the crab cakes in the hot oil to cook for 5 minutes or until the crab cakes are golden brown.
5. Serve immediately and enjoy.

Veggie and Quinoa Bowl

There is a reason why people have been raving over quinoa over the past few years. That's because there are a lot of undeniable health benefits that this gluten-free food provide. Quinoa is rich in protein (recognized as one of the most protein-rich foods), contains loads of fiber, plus other nutrients such as iron, lysine, magnesium, and manganese. If you're wondering if it can help you lose weight, well, yes it does! Because it is high in fiber, protein and has a low glycemic index, this food can help prevent hunger pangs, improve health, and aid in weight loss.

Ingredients:
½ cup quinoa, rinsed
1 cup low sodium vegetable broth
1 cup broccoli florets, roughly chopped
½ cup button mushrooms, sliced
1 tsp. coconut oil or olive oil
salt and pepper to taste

Steps:
1. Drizzle olive oil in a non-stick pan and heat over medium-high fire.
2. Throw in the chopped broccoli and sliced mushrooms. Stir and cook for 5 minutes. Turn off the heat and set aside.
3. Take a huge sauce pan and pour the vegetable broth and quinoa. Stir and bring to a boil.
4. When boiling, reduce the heat to low and then allow to simmer until most of the liquid is absorbed by the quinoa. Remember to stir once in a while.
5. When the quinoa is cooked, throw in the cooked vegetables and then season with salt and pepper.
6. Stir and cover. Allow to sit for a few minutes before transferring into serving bowls.
7. Serve warm. Enjoy!

Mexican Roll

If you're like me who loves Mexican food, then you'll surely love this recipe of the burrito.

Ingredients:
1 can (15 oz.) black beans
½ cup button mushrooms, sliced
1 pc. ripe avocado
1 small bell pepper, chopped
¼ cup onion, chopped
¼ cup spring onions chopped
¼ cup cilantro, chopped
½ tbsp. olive oil
4 pcs. whole-wheat tortillas
Sriracha sauce (optional)

Steps:
1. Thoroughly rinse the black beans and then drain. Set aside.
2. Drizzle the olive oil in a skillet and heat over medium fire. Throw in the chopped bell pepper, onion, and sliced mushrooms and sauté for a few minutes, or until the vegetables are tender.
3. Add the drained black beans into the pan along with the spring onions and cilantro. Stir and cook for 2-3 minutes.
4. Turn off the heat and set aside.
5. Remove the peel and pit of the avocado and place the meat in a bowl. Using a fork, mash the avocado until your desired consistency is achieved. (I like mine a bit chunky.)
6. Arrange the burrito by laying the (warm) whole-wheat tortillas on a plate. Scoop the black bean mixture on top and then a dollop of the avocado mash.
7. Roll up the burrito and serve with Sriracha sauce.
8. Enjoy!

Chicken Cutlets with Cherry Salsa

This family-friendly salsa is a must-try over chicken (even over baked tofu/ pork chops if you prefer) for a tasty, healthy dinner!

Ingredients:
Cherries: 1/2 pound, pitted
Extra-virgin olive oil: 2 tablespoons
Whole wheat breadcrumbs: 3/4 cup
Ground black pepper: 1/2 teaspoon
Ripe tomato: 1 large, cored, roughly chopped
White onion: 1/2 cup, chopped
Salt: 3/4 teaspoon, divided
Fresh cilantro (chopped): 2 tablespoons
Chicken cutlets (boneless, skinless): 4 (5 ounces each)

Steps:
1. Coat the cutlets with salt (1/2 teaspoon) and pepper (1/4 teaspoon). Place the breadcrumbs into a shallow, wide dish and dredge the seasoned chicken in breadcrumbs to coat. Transfer the coated chicken to a large plate after discarding and shaking off any excess crumbs.
2. Heat olive oil over medium high heat in a large skillet; add the cutlets arranging them in a single layer and working in 2 batches if needed; cook for 6-8 minutes, flipping once, until golden brown and cooked through. Transfer to plates
3. Place the onion, salt (1/4 teaspoon), pepper (1/4 teaspoon), cherries and tomato into a food processor, pulse until it turns into a chunky salsa. Add cilantro with stirring. Spoon this salsa over the top of the cutlets.

Tofu triangles with peanut sauce

This is a really tasty dinner option. Make sure to freeze/thaw/press the tofu as this will give the tofu a better, chewier texture.

Ingredients:
Firm tofu: 14 ounces, drained, sliced into 4 slabs (1" each)
Toasted sesame seeds: 2 teaspoons
Green onions: 4, finely chopped
Organic honey: 1 tablespoon
Natural peanut butter: 2 tablespoons
Peanut oil/sesame oil: 1 teaspoon
Soy sauce (reduced-sodium): 2 tablespoons
Rice wine vinegar: 1 tablespoon
Red pepper flakes: 1/4 teaspoon
Water: 1/3 cup

Steps:
4. Combine peanut butter, honey, half of the onions, soy sauce, vinegar, water and pepper flakes in a food processor; blend until smooth
5. Cut each tofu slabs into 2 triangles. You'll have a total of 8 pieces of tofu. Blot with paper towels.
6. Heat a sprayed pan on medium-high heat; add oil and heat it up; add tofu and fry, turning once until golden on both sides.
7. Add the prepared sauce to the pan; cook for few more minutes until bubbling.
8. Remove tofu from heat; top with remaining green onions and sesame seeds.

Kale Salad

This salad with its savory, sweet and spicy may be just what you are looking for.

Ingredients:
Organic kale: 1 bunch
Small sweet onion: 1/3, thinly sliced)
Organic cooked chickpeas: 1/2 cup of
Raisins: 1/3 cup
Organic sesame tahini: 1/3 cup
Cayenne or paprika: a pinch
Lemon juice: 1/2 cup
Salt: 1 teaspoon

Steps:
9. Mix the first 4 ingredients together.
10. Combine the rest ingredients separately as a dressing.

Cod with coriander & carrot pilaf

The unique spice blend utilized in this healthy dish converts plain frozen cod into a special dish you will enjoy yourself and can proudly serve to anyone.

Ingredients:
Olive oil: 2 tablespoons
Vegetable stock: 600ml
Carrots: 2 large, grated
Onion: 1, chopped
Chopped coriander: 2 tablespoons
Cod fillets: 4, skinless, about 175 g/6 ounces each
Lemon: 1, zest & juice
Cumin seeds: 2 teaspoons
Basmati rice: 200 g

Steps:
11. Heat the grill pan to high; use double thickness foil to line the pan; brush lightly with oil. Place the cod, lemon juice and zest, a little more oil and coriander

along with pepper and salt into the pan. Grill until the fish flakes easily, for around 10-12 minutes.
12. Heat the remaining oil in a separate pan and fry the cumin and onion for a few minutes. Stir in the carrots. Then add the rice with stirring until glistening. Add the stock and boil the mixture. Cover and cook gently until the stock absorbed and the rice is tender, for around 10 minutes.
13. Divide the rice onto 4 plates, place cod on top and pour over the pan juices.

Tips: While lining the pan, make sure to curl up the edges to catch the juices.

Veg Stir-Fry

The quick-cooking method of stir-fries retains both flavor and crispy texture and thus makes the most of lean proteins and lots of fresh vegetables. Since stir-frying is fast, you should have the ingredients prepped before cooking.

Ingredients:
Extra virgin olive oil: 1-tablespoon
Carrot: 1 medium, peeled & cut into thin sticks
Sugar-snap peas: around 100 g
Freshly ground black pepper
Asparagus tips: around 100 g
Tender stem broccoli: around 100 g, halved lengthwise
Runner beans: around 100 g, sliced
Balsamic vinaigrette: 4 tablespoons
Chopped fresh parsley
Salt

Steps:
1. Heat the oil in a large pan.
2. Add the carrot sticks and stir fry for a minute.

3. Add the runner beans and broccoli; stir fry for one more minute
4. Add the asparagus tips and sugar-snap peas; fry for a couple of minutes.
5. Add the vinaigrette with stirring, sprinkle with salt, pepper and parsley.

Mango Salsa & Salmon Tacos

Mix up your weekend barbecue with this savory recipe!

Ingredients:
Corn tortillas: 8
Arugula
For Fish seasoning
Fish: 1 pound (cod, halibut, salmon or tilapia)
Salt: ¼ teaspoon
Paprika: 1 teaspoon
Lemon juice: 1 teaspoon
Chili powder: ½ teaspoon

- For Chili Pepper Sauce:

Plain greek yogurt: ½ cup
Reduced fat mayonnaise: ½ cup
Lime: 1, zest and juice
Paprika: ½ teaspoon
Chili powder: ½ teaspoon
Oregano: ½ teaspoon
Jalapeño: ½, minced & seeded
Cilantro: 1 teaspoon, minced

- For Mango Salsa:

Mangos: 2 ripe, peeled and diced
Red onion: ¼ cup, diced
Red pepper: ¼ cup, diced
Chopped cilantro: 1 teaspoon
Lime: 2, zest and juice

Steps:
- For Fish

1. Combine chili powder, paprika, and salt in small bowl.
2. Preheat oven to 450°F.
3. Pat dry fish, sprinkle olive oil to lightly coat both sides of fish.
4. Place the fish on a tin foil lined baking sheet, keeping skin side down on the sheet. Sprinkle the fish with lemon juice and season with the herb mixture.
5. Bake for 12 to 15 minutes until fish is cooked through.
6. Break the fish apart into bite size pieces.

- For Chili Pepper Sauce

1. Place all ingredients in a medium bowl & stir until combined.
2. Store in the fridge.

- For Mango Salsa

1. Place all ingredients in a medium bowl & stir until combined.
2. Store in the fridge.

- For the tacos

1. Warm up tortillas in oven for 2-3 minutes at 450°F.
2. Arrange a layer of fish pieces onto tortilla, spread the sauce over fish, spread some arugula, and spoon mango salsa on top.

Salmon and Lemon

You do not have to be worried anymore with salmon recipes. I intended to put a couple of salmon recipes here all for you. Here's one with some lemon, capers, pepper, and everything healthy and nice.

Ingredients:

1 sliced thinly lemon
1 pc 32oz Salmon
1 pinch of salt and pepper (freshly ground)
Olive Oil (Drizzle)
1 tbsp thyme (fresh)
1 tbsp capers

Steps:
1. Place a baking sheet together with parchment paper and put salmon on top and remove skin.
2. Put salt and pepper on top of the salmon depending on desired seasoning quantity.
3. Place and arrange capers beside the salmon. Put the thyme with sliced lemon on top.
4. Place the salmon in the oven, then switching the setting to 400 degrees F.
5. Leave it there for 25 minutes and serve immediately afterwards.

Grilled Pork Loin Chops with Mustard Sauce

We all need proteins and a bit of fat from time to time, but we need to make sure that they are very healthy. We cannot sacrifice the progress that you have made, can we? Here is a recipe to support your progress and keep you healthy!

Ingredients:
4 portions Pork chops/ 2 tenderloins, or any preferred part
½ cup mustard
3 tbsp vinegar (raspberry or any mild vinegar alternative)
1 shallot or ¼ diced small onions
¼ cup oil (extra virgin)
¾ pounds apricots (6 pieces) No seeds and diced
¼ cup shredded basil
1 tsp. cardamom (optional)
Salt and pepper (for seasoning)

Steps:
1. Bring out the chops from the refrigerator and let it sit under 30 minutes to 1 hour (room temperature)
2. Season with salt and pepper then spread mustard all over.
3. Prepare the grill and preheat
4. Place all other ingredients in a medium bowl.
5. Toss and mix; add some salt and pepper if necessary for added taste.
6. Place chops onto the grill in medium to high heat for more or less 5-6 minutes on both sides.
7. Flip if there is visible grill marks on the each side. If you happen to have cuts with fats on them, be very careful on causing flare ups.
8. Brush the side with more mustard whenever you flip the meat.
9. Place the chops on your serving plates and serve.

Note: Better to serve the chops with salad on the side. You can make grilled asparagus and mushrooms as a grilled salad to compliment the meal.

Home Made Shepherd's Pie

This shepherd's pie is calibrated well for your diet. Though, yes, it has a long list of ingredients, you will never want to have another style of shepherd's pie after you've tried this.

Ingredients:
4 cloves minced garlic
2 chopped carrots
1 can 60oz tomato paste
1 medium yellow onion
2 lbs ground beef (grass fed)
1 container 8oz sliced mushroom
2 tbsp thyme
½ cup coconut milk
1 tbsp butter and additional bits as extra
1 tbsp chopped fresh rosemary
1 bag thawed peas (frozen)
2 tbsp balsamic vinegar
4-6 sweet potatoes (medium)
Salt (Natural Sea) and Pepper (Freshly Ground)

Steps:
1. Prepare the oven for 350F
2. Using a large skillet, saute the meat with garlic and butter.
3. When meat becomes brown, lift it from the pan. Place onions, mushrooms and carrots. Check it until the onions become transparent and carrots become soft.
4. Put the meat back to the pan. Then pour in the balsamic vinegar, thyme, tomato paste and a pinch of salt
5. Leave everything until the liquid dries out from the skillet.
6. Put in the peas and stir.
7. Place all the cooked meat into a 9x13" baking dish.

8. Place the sweet potatoes in a foil lined baking sheet and bake it until it becomes soft, approximately 40 minutes, depending on the size of the potatoes used. You can do this step while simultaneously cooking the meat)
9. Let the sweet potatoes cool down for a number of minutes. Peel open and place it together with butter, coconut milk, salt and pepper in a medium bowl.
10. Make a mash out of the sweet potatoes then spread it into the mixed meat.

NOTE: Having a finished uncooked pie baked in the oven for about 15-20 minutes. Wait until the center is hot and the sides are having bubbles on it.

Tomato and Onion Shrimp

Let's include some seafood in our daily diet. Meat and pork aren't the only things that can give you good health. Expand your horizon when it comes to food and try to appreciate what mother earth can give you from the natural waters!

Ingredients:
    1 pound large shrimp; frozen (approx.. 21-25 /lb)
    1 tbsp of your favorite blend spice
    3 tbsp fat (you can use your preferred kind)
    ½ cup tomatoes (cherry; washed)
    1 pc whole lime
    1 pc onion (sliced thinly)
    Salt (Kosher) for adding taste

Steps:
1. Defrost bag of shrimp in cold water until fully thawed

2. After thawing, dry shrimps using kitchen towels, then place it all in a bowl. Season them with your favorite spice blend.
3. Grab a skillet, then melt on a medium heat a tablespoon of fat.
4. Put in some salt and pepper; add some onions and wait till it becomes caramelized and translucent or transparent
5. Put in the tomatoes with the melted fat. Wait until it gets warm. So not wait for the tomatoes to pop or explode.
6. Lift the tomatoes together with the onions off the pan.
7. To make way for the shrimp, add some more fat onto the medium heat skillet.
8. Sautee the shrimp. Divide it into two parts and cook each side for a minute.
9. Check if the shrimp is fully cooked.
10. Put the sautéed onions and tomato on top of the shrimps
11. Squeeze the lime to top the dish off
12. Serve it hot

Pistachio Crusted Salmon Dinner

Nuts are good for your brains and health. Pistachio tastes good to, and if you haven't tried including it in your diet yet, here is the chance to try it. Let us match it with salmon to add a little punch to your dish!

Ingredients:
1 lb salmon fillet (deboned with skin)
3 tbsps mustard (preferably whole grain)
½ cup pistachios (salted and crushed)
Salt (Kosher) for seasoning
1 tbsp chives/scallions (chopped)
Pepper (freshly ground)

Steps:
1. Prepare the oven being preheated at 400 Degrees F
2. Grab a parchment paper on a baking tray
3. Using a paper towel/kitchen towel, remove excess liquid from the salmon and slice the salmon in 3 equal sizes
4. Place the chives/scallions and mustard in a bowl and mix them
5. Spread the mixture on top of the salmon
6. Using the crushed pistachios, drizzle it on top of the mustard topped fish and make sure to press it gently, assuring it to stick properly.
7. Put the marinated fish into the oven for 10 minutes or until the fish would reach the preferred doneness. If thinking of increasing the size of the fish into 1 pound, also increase the length of baking to 15 minutes
8. Put out the baked salmon and let it sit for a few minutes.
9. Serve with vegetables if you want.

Asian Style Grilled Chicken

We are now done with pork, meat, and seafood. Let's try white meat this time and grill it so we can avoid the extra cholesterol that frying can give to us.

Ingredients:
2 cloves garlic (minced)
3 tbsps vinegar (rice wine)
1 tbsp fish sauce
1 bunch scallions (cut and trimmed 1/3 size)
8 slices ginger (approx. ¼ size)
1 tbsp coconut aminos
½ tsp sesame oil (toasted)
4 lbs chicken (thigh)
2 tsps salt (Kosher)
2 tbsps honey (alternative: ½ small apple; peeled, diced and cored)

3 tbsps oil (macadamia) (alternative: preferred fat)
Pepper (Freshly ground) for additional taste

Steps:
1. Place some ginger, scallions and garlic onto the blender
2. Also put some of the other stuff into the mix to add to the marinate such as the vinegar, macadamia nut oil, coconut aminos, honey, sesame oil, pepper and kosher salt
6. Blend until smooth and even
7. Place the chicken parts into a bowl
8. Pour in the blended marinade onto the bowl and spread it all throughout the chicken.
9. Place it in the refrigerator for the mix to soak in nicely to the chicken for up to 12 hours.
10. Put out the chicken from the refrigerator and start the oven preheating at 400 degrees F
11. Place a foiled baking sheet or a wire grated rack onto the oven. Arrange the parts in such a way as the chicken's skin is facing up. Avoid having too much marinade still attached to the chicken or else it may become soggy.
12. Bake the chicken for a time of 40 minutes.
13. Make sure to flip the chicken halfway the cooking process to make the baking cooked evenly
14. A sign if the chicken is ready when the skin becomes crispy and golden brown. It would also be ready when the temperature would reach 165 Degrees F
15. Serve Immediately while it is hot.

Chapter 4: Snack and Dessert Recipes

Tell me about a person who doesn't love snacks and dessert, because that is just unbelievable. Snacks help fuel your system between meals. Healthy snacks keep your fat-burning metabolism accelerated. Here are some healthy snacking choices that will assist you reach your weight-loss goals and satisfy your diet cravings. Since we are all so addicted to snack and dessert, here are healthy recipes to save you from getting extra weight and unhealthy body!

Cinnamon popcorn

Avoid eating unhealthy popcorn at the movie theater. Follow the recipe to make your own healthy snack with lots of flavor and without any added fat. Plus it only takes 5 minutes to prepare!

Ingredients:
Popcorn: 100g
Ground cinnamon, : ½ teaspoon
Light olive oil: 2 tablespoons
Salt: A large pinch

Steps:
1. Take a medium size pan with a tight fitted lid.
2. Place all four ingredients into the pan; stir thoroughly.
3. Cover with the lid; heat gently, shaking every now and then. You'll hear the kernels popping.
4. Remove from the heat when the popping sound subsides. Let it sit until the popping sounds have stopped.
5. Remove the lid and stir thoroughly to keep the popcorns from burning at the bottom
6. Let it sit to cool slightly before serving.

Hormone Trail Mix

This delicious recipe is simple to make, and is packed full of fiber, both insoluble & soluble, which boosts healthy gut flora and digestive function. The dish will espccially be a lifesaver when you're busy or when you'll want a quick, high-protein meal at your desk.

Ingredients:
Roasted sunflower seeds: 15 ounces
Toasted, flaked coconut : 6 ounces
Almonds: 7 ounces
Raw pumpkin seeds: 15 ounces
Dried cherries: 6 ounces

Steps:
Toast necessary ingredients
Mix together in bowl.
Store in Tupperware.

Gingersnap Oatmeal

Have this snack with 1/2 cup milk for a complete evening snack.

Ingredients:
Quick-cooking rolled oats: 1/4 cup
Gingersnap cookie: 1, coarsely crushed

Steps:
Follow the package directions to cook the oats.
Sprinkle with the gingersnap cookie.

Granola bars

This healthy and deliciously easy all natural granola bars is great for snacking on the go.

Ingredients:
Slivered almonds: 2 tablespoons
Dried apricots: 1/4 cup, chopped or other dried fruit
Traditional rolled oats: 1 1/4 cup
Organic honey: 1/4 cup
All natural peanut butter: 1/4 cup (chunky or regular)
Vanilla extract: 1/2 teaspoon
Dried cranberries: 1/4 cup
Raw sunflower seeds: 2 tablespoons
Sesame seeds: 2 tablespoons

Steps:
1. Melt the honey, peanut butter and vanilla on high for 45 seconds, stir.
2. Place the rest ingredients in a separate bowl & mix; add peanut butter mixture with stirring; combine the mixture well.
3. Spoon the mixture in a non-greased 8" square pan; bake for 10- 15 minutes at 350° until light golden brown.

Smoked Paprika Almonds

Here is a fun little cocktail snack that is high in protein and quite tasty.
Ingredients:
Olive oil: 2 tablespoons
Cayenne: ¼ teaspoon
Sea salt: 1 teaspoon
Raw almonds: 3 cups
Garlic: 2 cloves
Smoked paprika: 2 teaspoons

Chili powder: ¼ teaspoon

Steps:
1. Heat oil over medium heat in a large skillet.
2. Add garlic; sauté until the garlic is almost brown, for 3-5 minutes.
3. Add the salt, cayenne, smoked paprika and chili; make a paste with stirring.
4. Add the almonds; stir constantly to coat them thoroughly with the paste.
5. Continue toasting the almonds for about 5 minutes more until they are fragrant.
6. Remove from heat; let sit to cool in the pan.

Veg chips

Simply create your own crunchy snack just by using veggies!

Ingredients:
Eggplant: 1 medium
Olive oil
Beets: 2 medium
Carrots: 2 large
Yam: 1 medium
Turnips: 2 medium
Dried herbs of preference such as cumin, oregano, ginger

Steps:
1. Preheat oven to 250°F.
2. Cut the vegetables lengthwise into ½ pieces.
3. Place the vegetables on wire rack on top of baking sheet; bake for around 1 hour, ensure even cooking by checking and turning 2/3 times.
4. Remove from oven when crisp, let sit to cool.
5. Sprinkle with spices.

6. Tips: If you're eating right away, drizzle the chips with oil. Store the remaining for up to 1 week in air tight container.

Toasted coconut cereal

This is an easy, four ingredient coconut dish that you can enjoy with some coconut milk in the evening. Time to start including this healthy cereal into your snack rotation!

Ingredients:
Unsweetened coconut flakes: 3 ½ cups
Swerve: 4 tablespoon
Cinnamon: 1.5 tablespoon
Grass-fed butter: 2 tablespoon

Steps:
1. Melt the butter along with the Swerve and cinnamon over a low heat.
2. Place the coconut into a bowl and pour over the butter mixture with stirring; spread the mixture over a lined baking tray.
3. Cook in an oven preheated to 340^0 F for 5-6 minutes. To prevent burning, stir and flip every few minutes.
4. Let it sit to cool; serve with coconut milk.

Blueberries & Goat Yogurt

Goat yogurt? Have you let yourself try one yet? It is healthier than your plain old yogurt and here is a recipe to not only improve your first experience with it, but help you reset your hormones too! It is unbelievably quick and easy, try it!

Ingredients:
1/2 banana (frozen)
1/2 cup blueberries (frozen)
1/2 cup of water
1/2 cup of goat yogurt (plain)
1 tbsp. of chia seeds
1 serving of whey protein isolate

Steps:
1. Simply place all six ingredients in a blender.
2. Puree, preferably high, until smooth and serve.

Tulsi Gelatin

Gelatins are undeniably good for both snacks and desserts. Kids love them and adults too. Here is a recipe for tulsi gelatin that can give you your gelatin fix without having to worry about the sugar. I hope you enjoy it!

Ingredients:
3 bags tulsi tea
1 tbsp honey or ¾ stevia (liquid)
2 cups water (very hot)
4 tbsp gelatin (grass fed)
1 pound strawberries (organic; trimmed)

Steps:
1. Grab a medium sized bowl, pour the water together with the tea bags. Place it on the side and let the tulsi bag soak for about 8-10 minutes.
2. Mix in the strawberries in a blender. Make sure that is smooth and evenly blended.
3. Measures about a cup and a half of strawberry puree. Afterwards, grab a large bowl
4. and place it in together with the freshly brewed tea, gelatin and sweetener.
5. Place in a glass pan 8x8" or preferred mold.
6. Place it in refrigerator to let it harden and set.
7. Make square cuts out of the mold gelation and serve immediately.

Cinnamon Apple Chips

Everybody loves chips, who doesn't? However, we are aware about what it can do to our bodies. Still, whenever we go and watch a movie, we just can't help but buy one of those chips and indulge. No more worries, here is a new homemade solution for that!

Ingredients:
1 tsp. of cinnamon
2 apples

Steps:
1. Pre-heat your oven to 200 degrees.

2. Slice the apples as thin as you can and get rid of the seeds.
3. Line a baking sheet with parchment paper.
4. Carefully line the sliced apples on the baking sheet. Make sure to avoid having them overlapped.
5. Sprinkle the apples with cinnamon.
6. Place the baking sheet in the oven and bake it for an hour.
7. Flip and continue baking for about an hour and a half.
8. Do not forget to flip from time to time until you do not see moisture on the sliced apples.
9. Store in an airtight container. Enjoy!

Almond Chia Pudding

I cannot stress anymore how good chia seeds are, some people are just crazy for them that they even make various dishes all with chia seeds. Want one? Here you go. Enjoy it as a pudding!

Ingredients:
3/4 cup of almond milk
3/4 cup of low-sugar fruit (raspberriess, kiwi, blueberries, kumquat)
1 tsp. Vanilla
1 ground cinnamon (sprinkle)
2 tsp. Honey
3 tbsp. of chia seeds (regardless of color)
Tapioca

Steps:
1. Mix the milk, vanilla, honey, and cinnamon in a medium-sized bowl.

2. Let the mixture sit in the fridge for a night until you see the chia seeds expand.
3. Finally, layer the chia mixture with tapioca in a glass.
4. Add fruit and enjoy!

Gummy Jellies

Everyone loves jellies, but most of us are worried about their sugar content and not so friendly food coloring. So what do we do? Below is a recipe to replace that worry-field previous recipe of jellies.

Ingredients:
1/2 tbsp. Natural orange flavor
1 tsp. of vanilla extract
1 pinch of sea salt
1 can of coconut or almond milk
1 1/2 tsp. of liquid stevia
1 1/2 cup of water
8 tbsp. of grass fed gelatin
Ice cube molds or fun-shaped ice molds

Steps:
1. In a bowl heat the coconut or almond milk and water over low heat.
2. Wait until it simmers.
3. Still over low heat, carefully add tablespoons of gelatin one by one.
4. Do not forget to mix while adding, until you do not see gelatin clumps anymore.
5. Carefully pour into the ice cube molds.
6. If there are excess mixtures, pour into a large glass pan.

7. Place both containers in the fridge and wait until they are solid.

8. Once solid, simply pop out of the mold and enjoy!

Eggs in Cups

Eggs are good for the body, even if you eat them everyday. They make you feel full quickly and can get rid of that snack craving in a couple of seconds. If you like them fried, just make sure that you stay away from vegetable oil, that's a killer. Enough with the oil reminders, here is a little recipe for a snack.

Ingredients:
4 tbsp. of cream (reduced fat)
4 tbsp. Parmesan cheese (grated)
4 eggs (whole)
4oz cheese (grated, reduced-fat)
8 strips of turkey bacon (cooked, finely chopped)
Cooking oil spray
Salt
Pepper

Steps:
1. Start by preheating the oven to 180 degrees C.

2. Layer the sides and bottom of four cups in a muffin tin with your oil spray.

3. Fill the four cups with chopped turkey bacon and grated reduced-fat cheese evenly.

4. Break an egg and add it to each cup.

5. Add some pepper and salt to the reduced fat cream and mix well.

6. Now add a tablespoon of cream to each cup.

7. Sprinkle some grated Parmesan on top of each cup.

8. Place the muffin tin in the oven and let it bake for 10 minutes.

9. Serve while warm. Enjoy!

Chapter 5: Smoothies Recipes

Nowadays, most of us are busy and we cannot afford to even sit on our dining tables to enjoy our food. Let's admit the fact that once we turn to full-blown adults, we forget everything else, except our busy career lives. Still, that is not an excuse to forget our health. No matter how busy we are, we should find a way for our health. While no money can mean no lifestyle, always remember that no health means no life, no lifestyle, and no money. Here are some smoothies to make our day right!

Mojito Smoothie

This tart smoothie disguises healthy veggies with satisfying mojito like taste! You can have this as a morning snack with yogurt or nuts on the side.

Ingredients:
Ice cubes: 3 cups
Water: 1/2 cup
Fresh mint leaves: 10
Orange: 1, peeled and segmented
Crushed pineapple: 1 can (7 ounce)
Baby spinach leaves: 2 cups
Banana: 1, broken into chunks
Lemon: 1, juiced
Lime: 1, juiced

Steps:
1. Place all nine ingredients in your blender.
2. Turn on the blender and process 'till nice and smooth.

Apple Mango Spinach Smoothie

Blend your way to health and wellness with this delicious smoothie.

Ingredients:
Plain Greek yogurt: 3/4 cup
Spinach: 1/2 bunch
Apple: 1
Mango chuncks: 1/2 cup
Ice/water: 1 cup
Protein powder: 1 scoop

Steps:
1. Place all six ingredients in your blender.
2. Turn on the blender and process 'till nice and smooth.

Nectarine Mango Smoothie

Boost your metabolism with this protein rich smoothie!

Ingredients:
Mango: 1, peeled & chopped
Water: 1/2 cup
Greek yogurt: 1/2 cup
Nectarine: 1, peeled & chopped
Protein powder: 1 scoop
Lemon rind: 1 teaspoon, grated
Ice cubes

Steps:
3. Place all seven ingredients in your blender.
4. Turn on the blender and process 'till nice and smooth.

Healthy smoothie

Jump-start your morning with this energizing, satisfying smoothie.

Ingredients:
Banana: ½
Apple juice: 1/2 cup
Mixed berries: 1 cup, frozen
Tofu: 1/4 cup

Steps:
1. Place all four ingredients in your blender.
2. Turn on the blender and process 'till nice and smooth.

Kefir Avocado Smoothie

Power yourself up with this delicious smoothie! You can make this smoothie even more protein-rich by adding spirulina, a protein rich super food that contains around 65 to 70 percent protein by dry weight.

Ingredients:
Kefir: 1 ½ cup
Avocado: ½
Plain Greek yogurt: ¾ cup
Chia seeds: 2 tablespoons
Goji berries: 1/3 cup
Gelatin: 1 tablespoon
Coconut oil: 1 tablespoon
Cinnamon: A dash
Optional
A little organic honey or stevia to sweeten
Spinach or kale: 1 cup
Berries (fresh or frozen): ½ cup
Spirulina : 1 tablespoon

Steps:
1. Place all twelve ingredients in your blender.
2. Turn on the blender and process for around 30-45 seconds 'till nice and smooth.

Frosty Summer smoothie

This pretty & pink frothy treat will cool you off on hot summer afternoon.

Ingredients:
Coconut water: 1 ½ cups
Lemon juice: 2 tablespoons
Protein powder (unflavored)
Frozen peaches: 1/3 cup
Frozen strawberries: ½ cup
Ice: 3/4 cup
Optional: mint leaves

Steps:
Place all seven ingredients in your blender.
Turn on the blender and process 'till nice and smooth.

Green Smoothie

This blended green smoothie contains fresh, whole fruits that will assist you in reversing some of the diet and lifestyle problems that worsens weight gain problem.

Ingredients:
Almond milk (unsweetened): 8 ounces
Avocado: ½ small
Spinach: 2-3 cups (or any green. I use kale and arugula too)
Banana: 1 medium, peeled

Steps:
1. Place milk and spinach in your blender and process 'till nice and smooth.
2. Add the banana and avocado, process for few more minutes until the smoothie gets a thick consistency.

Smoothie Very Berry Much

If there is one thing that our bodies can say to us after we drink this smoothie, it's this: "Smoothie very, berry much!" With the daily torture we do to our bodies, stress, improper eating, and lack of sleep, it's about time that we give it a treat and continuously do it.

Ingredients:
1/2 cup of blackberries
1/2 cup of raspberries
1 1/2 scoops of Daily Protein Strawberry flavor
3/4 cup of almond milk

Steps:
1. Make sure that your blender is clean.
2. Place all the ingredients in the blender.
3. Process until the mixture is smooth.

4. Add ice and enjoy!

All-In Banana Smoothie

Banana can do wonders to our skin, it provides us with potassium that our body needs for energy. Almond is good for our hormones and hemp seeds too. This smoothie is just packed with almost everything that you need for your hormone reset and it will give you energy too. It's yummy on its own way without the help of sugar.

Ingredients:
1/2 cup of almond milk
1 tbsp. of hemp seeds
2 pcs. Bananas (frozen)
2 tsp. maca
2 tsp. lemon

Steps:
1. Make sure that your blender is clean.
2. Place all the ingredients in the blender.
3. Process until the mixture is smooth.

Radish Smoothie

The lovely white radish and its nutritious leaves are packed with iron, calcium, magnesium, vitamin a, folate, vitamin c and vitamin k. One thing that they have in common is the effect that they have for your metabolism. Add apple, cucumber and lemon with that. Your body will just beam with pride!

Ingredients:
1/2 peeled lemon
1 apple (green)

1 cup of water
2 radishes including greens (small)
2 pcs. of cucumbers

Steps:
1. Make sure that your blender is clean.
2. Place all the ingredients in the blender.
3. Process until the mixture is smooth.

Strawberry and Chia Smoothie

Strawberries are packed with antioxidants and chia seeds are a good source of omega-3 fatty acids. That's hormonal balance, stronger immune system, and lovely flavor in one!

Ingredients:
1 tbsp. of chia seeds
1 cup of coconut water
2 pcs. Pitted dates
2 cups of strawberries (pitted)

Steps:
1. Make sure that your blender is clean.
2. Place all the ingredients in the blender.
3. Process until the mixture is smooth.

Green and Lean Smoothie

It rhymes and it is nice too! It's been said that greens, when it comes to diet, is never bad. If you are having a problem chewing those greens, drink them!

Ingredients:
1 cup of almond milk
1 banana (frozen)

1 date
1 cup of green tea powder
1 tsp. of vanilla extract
1 capsule of Wellness Resources green tea extract
2 organic peaches (medium)

Steps:
1. Make sure that your blender is clean.
2. Place all the ingredients in the blender.
3. Process until the mixture is smooth.

Flavored Popeye Smoothie

Almost everyone know who Popeye is. We can also say that his strength and health is because of his unending munching of spinach. While munching spinach is perfectly fine, wouldn't it be better if you drink it instead and add fun flavors to it?

Ingredients:
1/2 cluster of spinach
1/2 cup of mango (in chunks)
3/4 cup of Greek yogurt (plain)
1 apple
1 cup ice
1 scoop of protein powder (unflavored or vanilla)

Steps:
1. Make sure that your blender is clean.
2. Place all the ingredients in the blender.
3. Process until the mixture is smooth.
4. Add ice and enjoy!

Conclusion

Thank you again for downloading this book!

I hope this book was able to help you plan your diet carefully and in the healthy way that matches your diet well.

I encourage you to try the recipes I shared with you and you will realize that dieting, losing weight, healing your hormones, and being healthy is not synonymous to skipping meals or eating bland food.

From time to time, you might find yourself still staring at fast food and junk foods. Well, you are free to give yourself a treat at least once or twice a month. However, I must remind you that achieving your health goals is a matter of staying commited to the diet and embracing it as your new found lifestyle. You might not see the effects yet, but in the long run you will not regret it.

Boost your metabolism, reset your hormones, shed fat, and be ultimately healthy with through healthy foods. Happy eating!

Finally, if you enjoyed this book, then I'd like ask you for a *small* favor. Would you please take a minute or two to leave a review for this book on Amazon! Or you can go to this link:

This feedback will help us continue to write the kind of Kindle books that help you get results. And if you loved it, then please let me know.

Printed in Great Britain
by Amazon